Standing Together
Against
CANCER

40 Ideas to Support Your Loved One

Zana Kenjar

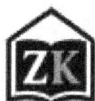

ZK PUBLISHING
HOUSE
A Home for Authors and Their Stories

Standing Together Against Cancer:
40 Ideas to Support Your Loved One

Copyright © 2025 Zana Kenjar
All rights reserved.

Published by ZK Publishing House,
Lincoln Park, New Jersey.

Previously published as In Search of the
Miraculous Cure (© 2022 by Zana Kenjar).

Macedonian edition published by Bata Pres,
Skopje, 2025.
Translated by Dr. Natasha Garrett.

Library of Congress Control Number: 2025922017

ISBN: 979-8-9987675-0-0
Printed in the United States of America

For media, rights/permissions, or bulk sales, contact:
Zana Kenjar
zana.kenjar@gmail.com

DEDICATION

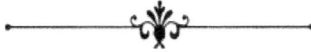

I dedicate this book to my younger brother Baskim.

"To the warrior, that defeats everything that comes his way with his positivity."

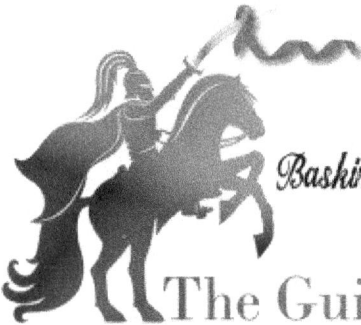

Baskim the Warrior

The Guiding Light

DISCLAIMER

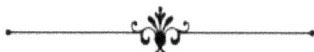

This book's purpose is to educate, inform, instruct and entertain. While it should be helpful, no book can tell you everything that you want to know or need to know about the topics it tries to cover. This book is not intended as a substitute for the medical advice of physicians, it's authors suggestions, ideas and opinion.

The reader should consult a physician in matters relating to his/her health with respect to any symptoms that may require diagnosis or medical attention. The author will not be held liable or responsible for any actual or perceived loss or damage to any person or entity, caused or alleged to have been caused, directly or indirectly, by anything in this book.

INTRODUCTION

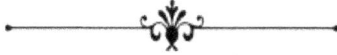

I've always known I wanted to write someday. There was always a yearning to leave something behind for my child and my family as a remembrance of me and my life. When it came time to doing so, I couldn't finish the book that I had been writing for the past few months. I was dealing with something very emotional and dear to my heart.

For the last 2 years, taking care of my brother has been the biggest concern for my family. Baskim was diagnosed with stage four lung cancer at the age of 45. This was the hardest emotional, physical, and mental journey he had to ever walk through, but he has done it with amazing grace.

His biggest gift of all has been his ability to keep thinking positively even in the hardest time of his life. He is a true inspiration for anyone that has not only dealt with cancer personally or with a loved one, but anyone who has gone through anything difficult. In this book, I will share what my brother, myself and my whole family has overcome through these difficult times in hopes that even one person will read it and find it helpful in getting through a difficult time in their lives. I will detail the difficult medical journey that Baskim has had to experience and, with that, the way in which our spiritual lives have also shifted, changed, and grown.

I hope to show how, even though you may be in pain, there are still ways to find the positive and treat every day as the gift it is. Please know that you are all in my prayers, and I pray you can find it in your hearts to keep my family and me in yours.

PROLOGUE

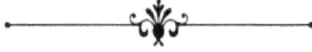

My Dear Reader,

I wrote my book in the month of Ramadan 2022. I signed up for coaching classes to learn how to publish my book, and my Great Coach Dennard Mitchell had a challenge for me and my partner, Jamez Morris, to write our books in 30 days.

I thought if my great coach for years helped authors write their books in 30 days, why couldn't I, especially in our beautiful month of Ramadan? I had a new strategy put in place. I was fasting during the day, helping my brother, taking care of my son, and cooking our dinners, all with the help of my husband. I would also write my book after we put our 6-year-old son to bed. The circle repeated for 30 days. I did it! I strongly believe that God is on this journey with us.

My Dear Reader, everything is possible when you put your mind to doing something you're passionate about. We are all capable of the impossible. Before I started my book, I imagined me holding it in my hands and reaching the entire world, reading and praying for my brother to get well.

Our mind is very powerful! Do what you love and go for it! Be your own king and queen of your hearts!

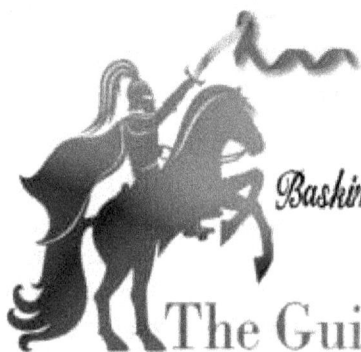

Bashim the Warrior

The Guiding Light

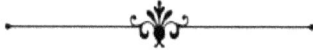

"Don't leave the sick alone. You will receive amazing blessings along the way!"

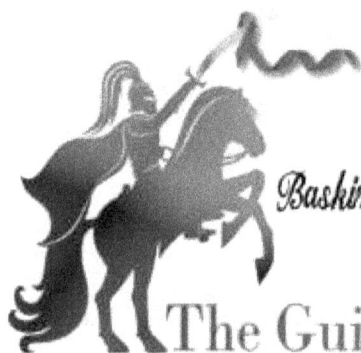

Baskin the Warrior

The Guiding Light

Table of Contents

ACKNOWLEDGEMENT

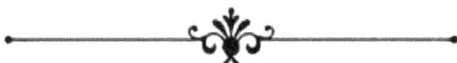

———————✦———————

I have been writing toward this goal for many years, and now I feel very appreciative to be the Author of this book. I would like to thank some people, among others, for their time and support along the path: to my dearest mother, Aniska Mustafoska, for loving me and supporting me unconditionally, to my younger brother Baskim Mustafoski, for his trust and allowing me to write about his journey, my amazing sister-in-law Ness Mustafoski for loving my work, my supportive brother Ramadan Mustafoski, my beautiful niece Leyla Mustafoski, her handsome fiancé Ned Bakic and his amazing family. To my handsome nephew Yasim Mustafoski for his support, to my husband Ned Kenjar and my beautiful son Sammy Kenjar for always cheering for me and being supportive. To song writer Elis for his support, to my beautiful friend Fatima Salkoski for her support, to my friend and neighbor Susan Mockler for her support, to my friend Jennifer Marks for her support, to my cousins and friends for their support. To my friend and Author Jamez Morris for her support. Special thanks to my coach Dennard Mitchell and his confidence in my ability to be an Author.

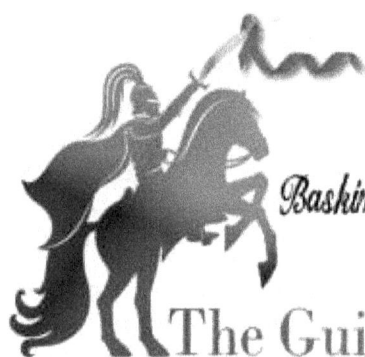

Bashim the Warrior

The Guiding Light

Chapter 1

THE DARK HOUR-
PANDEMIC AUGUST 2020

LOVING SUGGESTION #1

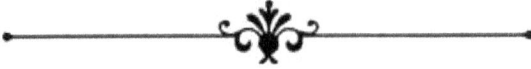

If a family member or a loved one has not been feeling well, encourage them to go to the doctor.

FAMILY CELEBRATION

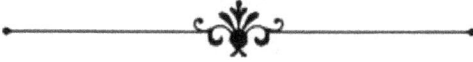

It was a beautiful August day
We were celebrating our holiday
Laughter, fresh foods, kids play
It was a perfect summer day

When I heard from your sweetheart
Pain has stroked you for some time
Waking and breathing were burdensome
And finally, we brought you in by force!

No words of comfort for weeks to come…

LOVING SUGGESTION #2

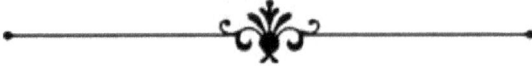

Never leave the sick alone in a hospital. Share their pain together.

Example: I had a schedule of who was going at what time each day, so he felt loved by many.

SHAKEN BY THE EARTHQUAKE

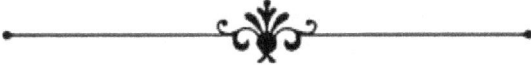

Waiting for weeks to hear good news
Walking the same steps as yesterday
White coats as they enter, the fear
Wishing for a glimpse of hope to be near

Our worries have not left us
Walking down through long hallways
Our bodies were tired but kept going
Weeks have passed dread was growing

Tired faces, only one allowed to enter
It was 2020; what a year!
Torment, Pandemic, everyone scared
Masked, waiting my turn to go inside

The young doctor entered, puzzled face
"Lung cancer," he said, "has spread."
Order in this courtroom, madness!
Confused, he replied, "I have Cancer?"

The pain has found its home ….

LOVING SUGGESTION #3

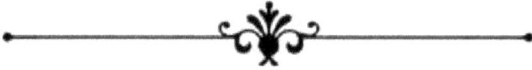

Even though you may feel defeated, try and pick up the pieces of you and those around you. Wipe your tears and try to help your loved ones stay in a good place. Have faith and be positive!

THE UGLY TRUTH

Perplexed, our hearts are raising
No, it can't be; we kept embracing
Our eyes are filled with countless tears
Fear of loss in older brother and sister

Each morning we face the truth
We want to go back to dreaming again
And thank God for another day
Yet, the ugly truth is here to stay

How can we all live this way?
He is convicted of pain every day
To fight an enemy hidden inside of him
Invisible, not tangible yet present, and real

What is the fairness in that?
Young body defeated by this demon
Will you fight him or will you surrender?
You said, "I'll fight till the last breath in me."

LOVING SUGGESTION #4

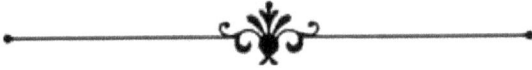

When trying to be supportive of a sick loved one, empathy is very important. Try to focus on their struggles when they are present and put yours aside for the time.

THE HEARTBREAK

Your love heard the devastating news
She knew what malignancy was
In her anguish and grief, a river of tears
But in front of you, she stood with no fears

Suffering from her own disease
Given a few months in this world
It's been fifteen years
Already they have shed so many tears

The sickness this young woman endured
It's tearing my heart into pieces
And the most heartbreaking was
Hearing her love has three months to live

"I won't accept, "she said. "I was told a few months."
"Here I am alive and he will be too."

The saddest thing I have ever seen...

LOVING SUGGESTION #5

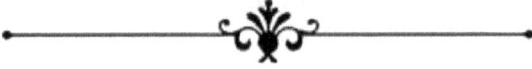

Trying to communicate a diagnosis to many different people in your loved one's life may be difficult for them. Sit down with them and try and come up with a way you can help them to do so, or make the announcement for them.

THE PATIENT

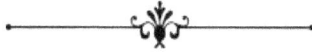

Living through torment and pain
Accepting the truth of his illness
Painful memories last a few months
Gray face, he has the look of a patient

Family calling around the globe
Grief, as I explain with a cracking voice
With each person, pain keeps repeating
Family crashed to the ground in agony

The mother feels his hardship inside
But the truth is never spoken to her
Only that her baby boy is a little sick
And not from the evil beast …

His love is near, suffering deeply
Forgetting her own pain, the deep wound
Both harmed; my heart is breaking
with disbelief, I silently weep inside, aching

Is this his destiny?

LOVING SUGGESTION #6

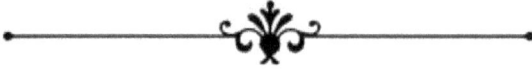

Daily prayer, meditation, affirmations and positive visualizations are key components to starting spiritual healing for the sick, as well as the individuals in their support system.

HEALING YOU ...

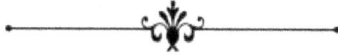

Oh brother, receive the fruits of my efforts
I lost myself, my hope, my mindset
I felt broken, lost, angry. Why you?
Will the sun be shining on us again?

Giving a helping hand each day
Nothing is worth saving anymore
When a loved one suffers so deeply
Figuring out how to be saved

I recite four healing prayers each night
For curing from our Prophet Mohamed
Oh, beautiful soul, may peace be upon you
Giving us hope with prayers so true

Using visualization, I wash the enemy
Clearwater runs through your body
Seven times, you are cleansed and pure
The light dissolves, disease washes away

We will find your cure!

LOVING SUGGESTION #7

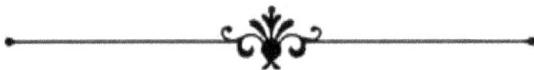

A mother's love is like nothing in this world. Protect your mom's feelings, especially when her child is suffering. As we say in Macedonia "the blessing is always under your mother's feet".

MOTHER'S VISIT

A few months have passed since she saw you
She hasn't felt his sweet embrace
She hasn't smelled her youngest scent
Her favorite youngest boy, her everything

As an observer shattering pain strikes me
I wonder if she knows if she feels his pain
She must have! the grey look, the face
And his bony body maneuvering slowly

She smiles and looks with love
He smiles back and embraces her
Hours of great times and laughter
Blessed, all her children have gathered

Oh mother, hope you never see the evil
And departing of your child first
There is an amazing beauty inside you
You look for love in everything!

I play your role in healing your son!

LOVING SUGGESTIONS #8

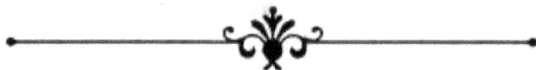

Time is the worst enemy when a loved one is diagnosed with a terminal illness. You wonder when their last breath is. We must find a place in our hearts to be strong for ourselves and our loved ones, beat fear, replace it with gratitude every day, and be happy. Make memories.

IS THE CLOCK TICKING ...

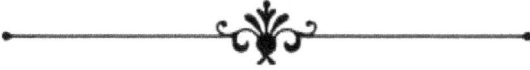

Time is the worst enemy now
As I look at myself in the mirror
Tomorrow is promised for none
Am I starting my day in despair?

I want to reset the clock to decades ago
Bringing you when you were twelve
We lived in faraway land next to a lake
So happy and healthy we played each day

Oh, father, you sold us the dream
Brought us to where dreams happen
Then from your limited belief, he fled
Found a new home and left…

Years passed, with a few minute's visits
Always waiting on holidays to be near
With disappointment on our faces
Another year, he was not here.

His love terminally ill before the wedding
For years of care, he felt a torment
I can't even imagine his heartbreak
And the daily fear of her departing

Oh, your soul, what have you endured.

LOVING SUGGESTION #9

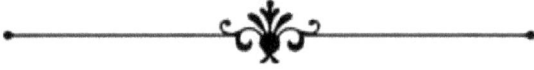

Acceptance is very difficult when a loved one is diagnosed with cancer. I struggled with accepting that my brother was so sick. What helped me is seeking guidance from a therapist. She told me I have to help myself before I help him, and suggested more sessions, meditation, exercise, affirmation and positive thinking. It helped me along the way.

GLIMMER OF HOPE

I want to pause the time
Make this an endless day
On your happiest day, so it doesn't end
As I break through this sadness I feel
And the heaviest rock I carry on my back
Can I feel the light again?
And laugh with happy tears
Do you remember our happy childhood?
I don't want us to be sad
I want to celebrate each day
You will be well and amongst us
For eternity!

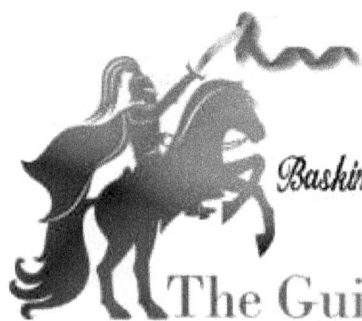

Baskim the Warrior

The Guiding Light

Chapter 2

IT'S NOT OVER, BEGINNING OF A NEW LIFE

LOVING SUGGESTION #10

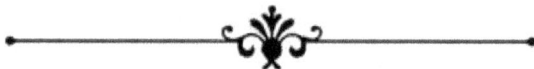

Give a positive light and a new way of life to the sick; help them start dreaming again.

TILL YOUR LAST BREATH

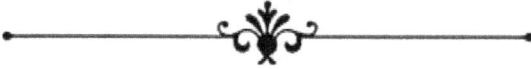

I will fight, as I looked up in the sky
I keep asking and asking why
But I am no stranger to change
New plans for you I must rearrange

I will bring an army to help
Don't want to see one tear shed
I will help pre-plan your daily life
And help you begin to strive

For months you have been inside
With your ill sweetheart by your side
The pain you both have shared
I haven't seen it anywhere

It's time for a walk to feel the sun

Loving Suggestion #11

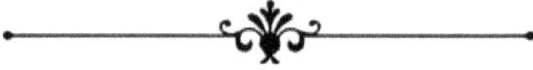

Being positive helps your heart feel joy again and your mind will find a solution.

POSITIVE TALKS

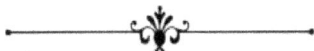

How do you communicate…
With the one with fresh broken wings
His tomorrow is not promised
The word "terminal" is so ugly to be honest

I will be the girl that's always been
Can't live in this space of agony
Positive talks are what I will choose
I won't believe any negative news

We will find the positive doctors!
The positive friends that love us
And the good neighbor that will help us
And create our own circle of trust

To God, we pray to bring us blessings today!

Loving Suggestion #12

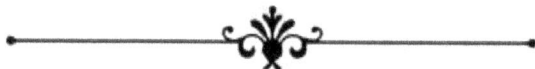

Visiting the sick is a blessing and a privilege; the visitor also benefits.

VISITING AND DAILY CARE

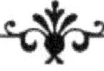

I wake up early and do Tony's prime
Meditation and daily prayer at the same time
Daily exercise keeps my body in shape
Affirmations run through my mind like a tape

After the school bus, I am headed there
Healthy breakfast for you to prepare
Organic greens, herbs and organic eggs
Great healing foods for you on that plate

Help you disinfect, so you live in a clean air
All clean rooms and your clothes you wear
Talking your clothes to wash is a pleasure
You guard your clothes like a true treasure

Always dressed up for every occasion
You should be a model instead of a mason!
May you enjoy your clothes in happy days
Traveling in linen pants and cool shades

LOVING SUGGESTION #13

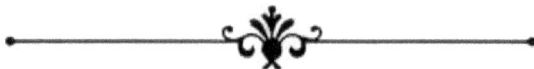

It's important to have a routine with calls and texts. I text my brother each morning to say hello and see what he feels like eating for breakfast and throughout the day.

DAILY CALLS AND TEXTS

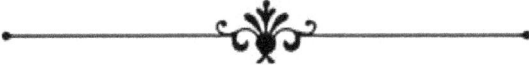

As I look for advice a wise woman said
don't text "how you feeling today"
Not healthy to feel like a patient every day
With cheerful voice, erase his gray day

I leave the day free for you to plan
Lunch, walk in the park and fresh air
With the intention of positive talk in advance
And leave future plans in your head to dance

LOVING SUGGESTION #14

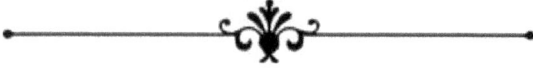

Include your loved one with dinner plans. See if they like to go shopping at their favorite food store. In addition, ask them if they can help you prepare the meal or find a good recipe.

WHAT'S FOR DINNER?

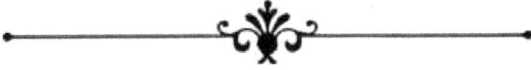

Reading what's the best foods to eat
Preparing each meal with love is a treat
Healing foods is always on the menu
And at times, we find a different venue

I dread the days when not in the mood
Then I think of your favorite food
Vietnamese soup will always get you out
I am liking the soup but not the sprouts

We found a great place for us to shop
Fresh foods galore for dinner each night
Organic chicken, fish or lamb is light
Amazing dinner on our table tonight

LOVING SUGGESTION #15

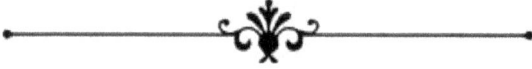

Include social life in their daily lives. Gather family and friends at least 1 to 2 times per month for tea or diners. Ensure it's on the calendar for all, and follow up a couple of days before with your guests if they are attending. This is very important for their psyche; they will feel life is still worth living.

FAMILY GATHERINGS

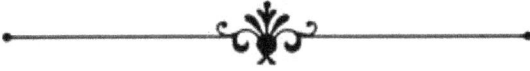

My Pre-plan is always my daily task
My iPhone calendar became my close friend
We gather close friends and family near
My main guest was always you, my dear

As we plan the foods, we bought to prepare
We think of the best clothes for us to wear
You enter and put your favorite music to play
We dance and sing our worries away

Serving desert is nephew's favorite time
Too much sweets are always a crime
To bring you a good time was a success
Hours passed, forgetting about the stress

With gratitude to God, we go to rest.

LOVING SUGGESTION #16

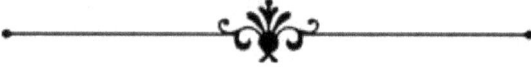

Resting is so much needed for the sick due to their physical limitations. Reach out with texts and phone calls to check in on them.

RESTING DAYS

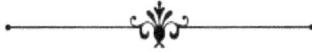

There are days you lay in bed all-day
This is the way you rest your body
Watching your cooking channel and shows
This is how your day goes

You love to feel the silence in your space
The doorbell rings with your favorite order
Even visitors are too much to see
In your own space, you want to be free

LOVING SUGGESTION #17

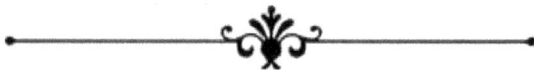

I believe the text at the end of the night is like a security blanket for the sick.

My brother gets very excited when I text him and wish him good night. He sends me cute emojis back.

END OF THE DAY, GOOD NIGHT

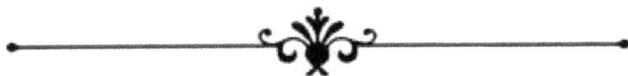

Texting at the end of the day to say good night
To surrender with no struggle or fight
Let your body rest and restore
Tell your mind to win the invisible war

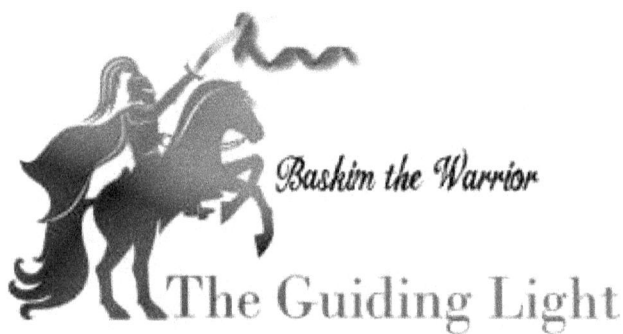

Baskim the Warrior

The Guiding Light

Chapter 3

THE MEDICAL HELP, HEALING YOUR HIDDEN WOUNDS.

LOVING SUGGESTION #18

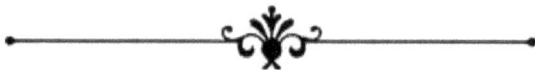

Before any scans be very positive and encourage your loved one to visualize the positive results ahead of time. If your loved one is not spiritual, pray for them and amazing results can happen.

Planning the Scans

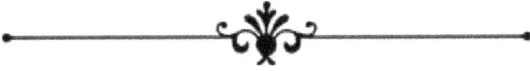

Praying and visualizing before the scans
That you will receive miraculous results
Visualizing the ugly demon is leaving
And freeing your soul from grieving

All the scans that you have done
Results brought us to a state of amazing joy
The demon was shattered and is shrinking
Great things happen with positive thinking

LOVING SUGGESTION #19

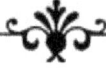

Doctor's visits are endless and exhausting with cancer patients. Some are weekly, while others are monthly, quarterly, and eventually annually. Arrange your schedule for the visit as best as you can. If you can't be there, coordinate with other friends and relatives to help out. Make sure to follow up with whoever is helping to ensure they are available the day or so before.

Depending on what is more comfortable or convenient for you, take notes during every visit. Ask friends and family to do so as well. Whether you use a note app or your phone, recording with video or sound or handwriting, make sure to organize all notes into one specific area, such as a separate hard drive. It may seem like a lot but staying organized has helped to quickly access the information later.

CANCER

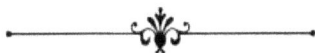

You are unwelcome intruder
Brought us pain and suffering
Our inner struggle is draining
Life hurts and we question
What to believe anymore …

Before this terror
If we knew, we'd been so lucky
But families had these days
I wasn't aware of how it cuts you
Unless you are in the fight

All my family broken
Didn't know you bombed us
How it's the same pain for all
Strange connection with sadness
It's love, maybe we are still lucky

He could have been alone!

LOVING SUGGESTION #20

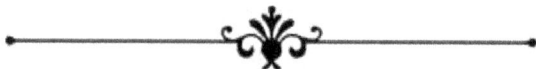

Choosing the right Oncologist is very important.
We were so impressed by Oncologist Dr. Stephan Dorkhom that we want the world to know of his amazing medical care and expertise.
Special thanks to Tiffany, Mellisa and Sharon.

Doc, this poem is for you!

THE ONCOLOGIST

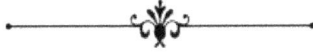

Doctor Dorkhom

Bless your parents for having you
And Blessed be till the end of you
The Monthly trip to your office is near
Dr. Dorkhom is here, no need to fear

You are Tony Robbins on steroids
Picturing your face on all the tabloids
For the world to know a true hero
No white coat can compete with what you know

Dr. Dorkhom, you are not just a cancer killer
But also, a human mind healer
And your positive and heartfelt grace
Never talked time in his face

Lifted his spirits and that he looks great
And that he will live and can still create
Follow through on all your promises
And you gave him his better days

All because of you, you gave him time

This journey is better with you!

LOVING SUGGESTION #21

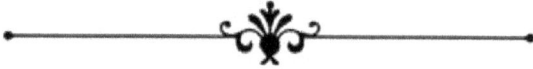

Choosing the right Nephrologist and the Dialysis Center is very important. It's their second home once your loved one starts dialysis treatments.

We were so impressed by Dr. Harjinder Saini and DeVita Dialysis Center in Wayne NJ, we want the world to know of their amazing medical care and expertise. Special thanks to Adrienne and Joselina.

Doc, this poem is for you!

THE NEPHROLOGIST

Doctor Saini

A decision had to be made
Spoke a long time to describe his state
Many sleepless nights to God, I prayed
The only option was the dialysis way

Doctor with a great bedside manner
And listened to our concerns for hours
Not your typical doctor but a good man
Years of making in this life span

Thanks to you, he has been healing
No more emergencies and crazy dealings
Results are better each week by week
Never seen a kidney doctor so unique

Dr. Thank you for saving my brother,

The journey is better with you!

LOVING SUGGESTION #22

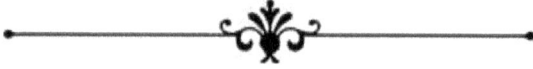

Choosing the right primary doctor is very important.

We were so impressed by Dr. Omar Nabulsi that we want the world to know of his amazing medical care and expertise. Special thanks to Dr. Jessica Chow.

Doc, this poem is for you!

YOUR PRIMARY DOCTOR

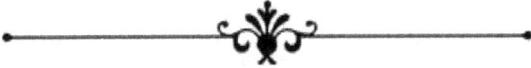

Doctor Nabulsi

Your knowledge and advice that you share
Your outstanding quality of medical care
Physical condition, straight from the gym
Or maybe you do hours of ongoing swim

Amazing office where everyone cares
Never waited long or had any despairs
Hey medical world, please be aware
He is a true example of primary care

Hospital visits, you ran to him every day
And complimented him in a great way
That he looks great and he will be ok
Your helping hand always found a way

Emergencies cases, and there were so many
Always by his side without any pride
Humble and caring doctor is what you are
To Baskim and Jen, you are the biggest Star!

Thank you for always taking time with him

This journey is better with you!

LOVING SUGGESTION #23

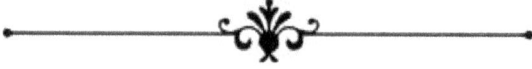

Choosing the right Vascular Surgeon is very important. We were so impressed by Dr. John Danks that we want the world to know of his amazing medical care and expertise. Special thanks to Margarita and Alice.

Doc, this poem is for you!

VASCULAR SURGEON

Doctor Danks

Second surgery is on the way

You were a hero from the start.
And didn't quit no matter what,
Your persisted to find a way.
To save my brother for a better day.

You saw inside his veins,
Miracles you are creating each day.
So many hours in the making,
Doctor, your reward is awaiting!

He stuck with you and said you care,
He said you loved the shirt he wears.
You showed him the same shirt in red,
Funny moments with you, I may add.

You have a personality like no other,
Excellent medical care for my brother.
A surgeon like you could never find.
Dr. Danks, you are one of a kind!

This journey is better with you!

LOVING SUGGESTION #24

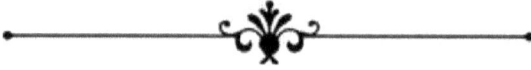

Prayer is important before surgery.
Stay with your loved one during the duration of the
surgery or arrange for a family member to help.

PRAYERS BEFORE SURGERIES

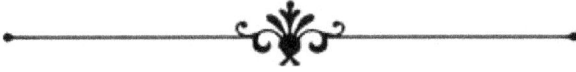

Asking God to keep you near
And not just for another year
Praying for decades to come
So, you can feel this amazing sun

You are so young and handsome
God had a plan in your making
All these obstacles are taken
There is a reason don't be mistaken

Prayers to be well

LOVING SUGGESTION #25

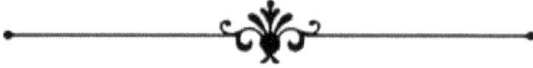

The power of thoughts can contribute to healing your loved one from suffering.

Send them video clips and other motivational materials to help keep positive thinking and thriving. Some I admire are: Tony Robins, Marisa Peer, Dr. Joe Dispenza, Abraham Hicks, late Louise Hay. I gave my brother a cube for listening to Joel Osteen. He plays the affirmation every day to start his day. It's important to find someone that speaks to your loved one in a positive way. This might not be a "motivational speaker." It could be a comic, a poet, an athlete, etc. Just find what works for them and keep sharing.

CHANGE THE LOVE FOR LIFE

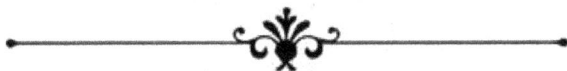

His storms didn't stop him from loving the sea.
He battled the storm and watched the waves
He changed his way of speaking
He changed his way of thinking
He doesn't feel that he is a victim
And he won't be a victim anymore
His thoughts created his experiences
And consciously created his thoughts

LOVING SUGGESTION #26

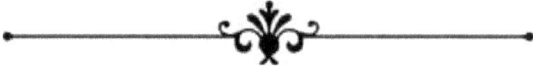

Hospital stays were very draining for my brother. A few things that helped were: staying in touch with him through daily calls, texts and group video chats.

THE HOSPITAL DAYS

We were away on a beautiful holiday,
Rooms were connected when you knocked.
Asleep, I answered if all were ok,
You said, "Not ok, we can no longer stay."

The hospital stays were so very frequent,
always needing some type of treatment.
Last one was the COVID, and was so scary,
Only daily visits from your primary.

You made a decision,
For Dialysis days to come into play.
There you started your treatment,
All alone as they didn't let us stay.

A new road of unfamiliar direction.

LOVING SUGGESTION #27

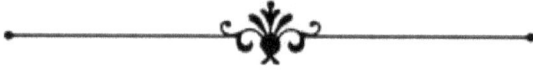

It's possible that starting dialysis treatments saved my brother. For my brother, it was Kidney failure due to complications from chemo, but whether your loved one is battling may often bring about unforeseen obstacles. It's important for you and them to take things one at a time. For me, it helped to concentrate on making my brother as comfortable as possible.

Currently, I take him to dialysis three days a week, and I wait for him with a warm car and blanket and food prepared or ordered to eat at home. I stay with him until he is ok and ready to rest. It's also helpful to get them ice pops. My brother loves them after dialysis session.

THE BEGINNING OF DIALYSIS DAYS

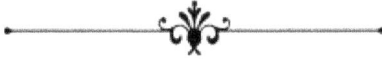

Your eyes were filled with nothing but sorrow
Each time I took you home
Your body was shaken and broken
As you looked for an escape from yourself

Long hours of cleaning your fluids
It has to be this way to live another day
The miracle is not far away; it's today
Don't stress; God's mercy is so amazing

I have been living with this thorn in my heart
It buried me alive in a grave of unhappiness
Waiting for a glimpse of hope your way
Praying dialysis days are not here to stay

LOVING SUGGESTION #28

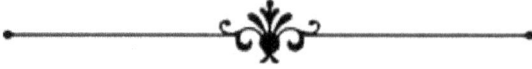

Don't give up hope for your loved one, even in their roughest times give them loving words and support them with their treatments. After 3 months of dialysis, my brother felt better, and his results were great. He no longer had to go to the emergencies for blood transfusion or needing hydration. All monitoring was conducted at the dialysis center.

I continue to support him and drive him for each session even though he can drive himself. There are still days that he feels broken, and I want to be there to pick him up and tell him it's okay.

ACCEPTANCE OF DIALYSIS AS DAILY LIFE

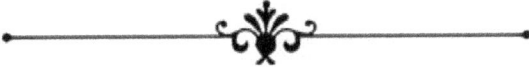

You rest the days when you are home
Only ten to twelve hours you spend at dialysis
It's only seven percent of the hours per week
The rest are your hours to live

Positive acceptance and smiles when we go
Don't see the grin and unhappiness anymore
Your desire to eat and thrive has come back
To take a drive with a snack in your hand

It has been four months or more
You haven't been a guest at the hospital
Your routine at dialysis was what you needed
With weekly care, the staff proceeded

You started to live all on your own
Cooking and playing your freestyle songs
My visits to cook are not so frequent
Each time I asked, you said you have eaten

Glimpse of hope to a great direction…

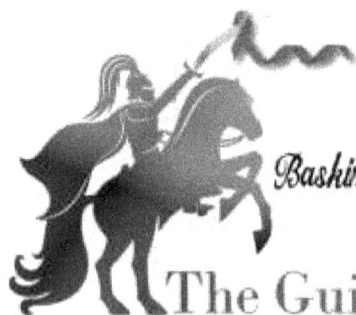

Bashim the Warrior

The Guiding Light

Chapter 4

ASKING PRAYERS FROM THE WORLD

LOVING SUGGESTION #29

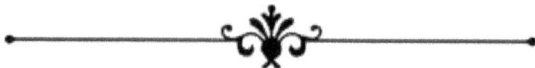

The benefit of prayer also goes to the person that prays for another. You will never know where the blessings come from.

Prayer from Around the World

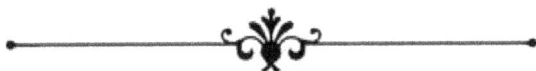

Oh, dear world, you are my office
I have traveled to many of your lands
Walked on your soils and your sands
Emersed in your nature with my bare hands

Oh, dear world
If you can only see inside my heart
My love is pouring above the charts
The blessing will be flowing in all your parts

I have an ask for each of you
And say a prayer for my brother
And to heal like no other
With all your hearts

Let's all start!

OH, HEALING TREES

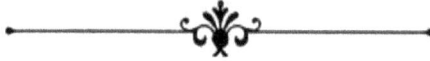

I always loved and painted trees
Using Bob Ross's techniques
Adding diversity to my yard's ecosystem
I am painting happy trees
Oak, pine, birch, and slippery elm trees
Bring him your medicinal properties
And natural healing remedies
Say a prayer for my brother
And for the miraculous cure
And give him oxygen galore
Let him feel your aura

CALLING ON THE SEA WORLD

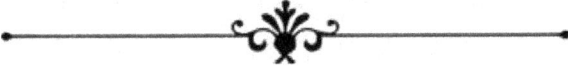

I swam in many seas
Oh, sea world, come and help us, please
My darling brother, assistance is near
Sea world is here, no need to fear

They'll give you the second chance you need
All gathered in the fastest of speed
Removed impurities while you dream
All working together as a true team

CALLING THE ANIMAL KINGDOM

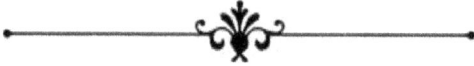

Hey Lion,
Calling on you, the one who
possesses kingship and leadership qualities
Gather your kingdom in all equalities
All shapes and sizes
Say a prayer for my brother
And rawer and cheer like no other

To All the Countries

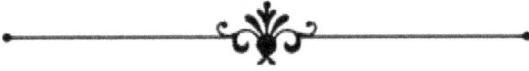

To all 195 countries in this world
With most beautiful scenic places
Intriguing architectures and history
And your colorful landscapes

You all have beautiful cultures
Use your natural wonders and faith
Say a prayer in your language
And kneel for him to heal

TO ALL THE INSECTS I FED

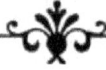

Oh, cute insects, you are so small
The fear in you because we're so tall
I helped you live in every season
Filled your bellies for that reason

I fed you daily my dinner crumbs
Happy gathered in an army of tons
I am asking you for all your blessings
To rise above from all your dwellings

Say a prayer for my brother

UNITED WE PRAY

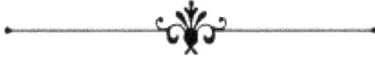

"The road to recovery "
If you have a brother, pray
If you have a sibling, pray
If you are saddened, pray
If you feel my pain, pray
If you are amazing, pray
If cancer ever touched you, pray
If you feel empathy for human life, say a prayer

TRIP TO JAPAN

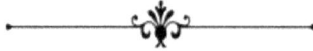

I will take you to Japan
Feed you the Waqyu steaks
And ask the cows to pray
And give you their energy
And great health today

HEY CELEBRITIES!

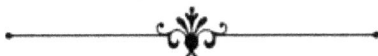

Celebrities on red carpers
Jlo, Beyonce, Oprah, Kardashians
You have a love like no other
The love for you and another
Gather your celebrity troops
And the rest of your groups
To say a prayer for my brother

TO ALL PLANETS

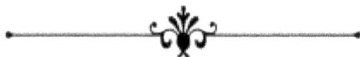

I am reaching out to you
From a faraway land
Please give me a helping hand
Send your prayers
For my brother

ALL COACHES AND SPEAKERS

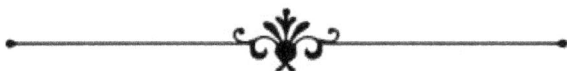

Joe, Tony, Marisa, Abraham, Bob
And many more I support each day
Forward my asking to all your fans
Touch the screens with your hands
Help me and say a prayer
For my brother

DEAR PRESIDENTS

To all the presidents
Past, present and future
In your G20 meetings
Instruct your countries
United, say a prayer
For my brother

OH STARS

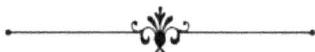

How beautiful you are
You who light up the sky
And bring life to the earth
When he is in the dark
Light up his day
And pray

OH SUN

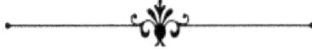

So big and bright
That gives us warmth
And light up our day
Give him healing energy
For a better day
And pray

All the Mosques, Churches and Temples

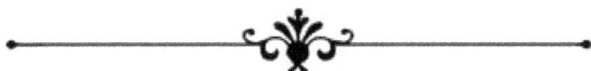

Oh, you, with teachings of the unseen world
Gather your good men who are heroes
And your faithful women as gentle as a rose
Innocent children whose prayer multiplies
And let this prayer rise

Let the unseen angels run to him
And cover him with blessings and love
And collectively, say a prayer from your heart
To find a cure and never be apart.

May your house of worship be glorious!

YOUR NEPHEW'S PRAYERS

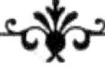

I am 6, and each night
I pray for you with my mom
I say God give my uncle
Second chance at life

To be alive forever
Buy me pizza for lunch
To buy me Legos and such
Uncle, I love you so much.

Praying for a miracle!

THE DESERVING OF YOU

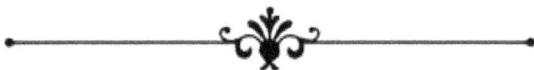

If I can…
I will place you in the Buckingham Palace
Rebuild it with pink star diamonds

Fly you to Spain to dine at the Sublimotion
With bright light, dissolve and end my mission
And bring you to your remission

I will carry you to Mount Everest
So, you can breathe the clean air
And the healing power of Nature

If I can't, God will find a way!

To All "You" That I Know!

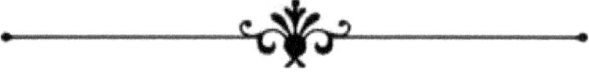

To all the people that I gave jobs
Helped you and healed your invisible scars
And lifted your spirits when you felt unjust

To all my former employees, leaders, CEO's
With my teachings and progress for 25 years
And made you successful in all your careers

To all my family and friends in Motherland
That I loved and helped over thirty long years
And prayed at night to remove all your fears

To all the doctors I have seen for decades
And I was loyal to you in all my stays
And all others I've touched in a positive way

Never asked for none, nor was I a seeker
In humility, I am asking for what is free
Pray for my brother in your highest decree

OH, PEOPLE WHO BECAME STRANGERS

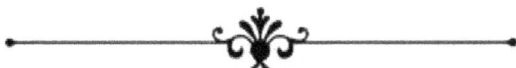

For all the people in any season
We left unspoken without a reason
Lessons learned, it's how we grow
Sharing one sky that fits us all

Diversity and Inclusion is what I know
Come inside through my open door
Say a prayer, and it's not a score
Welcome back, and don't ignore!

Say a prayer that's much needed
For a humble brother not conceited

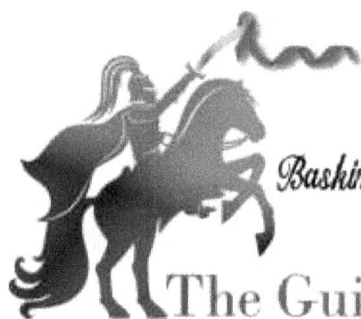

Bashim the Warrior

The Guiding Light

Chapter 5

MAKING MEMORIES

LOVING SUGGESTION #30

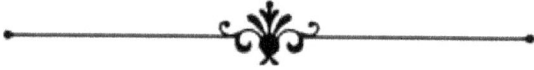

Keep planning trips and attending events with your loved one. It keeps them looking forward.

NIECE'S LEYLA ENGAGEMENT

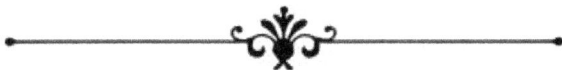

Snowy, icy day with doubt in our minds
Gathered together for a special night
You came, wanted to be by her side
"I am so happy for her," you replied.

Live music and happy folk songs
You were clapping and singing along
Authentic food for all of us to enjoy
Dancing, perfect night, what a joy!

LOVING SUGGESTION #31

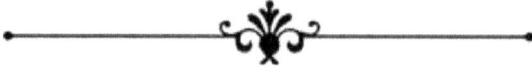

In my plans, I included short trips for something to look forward to; call the place you're going to ahead of time to make sure the area can accommodate special needs.

HAPPY SHORT TRIPS

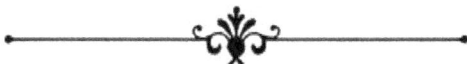

Monthly trips were so much needed
We packed our car, and we proceeded
To a special place called The Ocean
To escape daily struggles and emotion

You loved your room with a glass view
Sitting and staring at the waters so blue
Amazing lunches and dinners were awaiting
Beautiful memories we were creating

You watched our son so we can play free
The most precious moments spent with him
You are foody, and so is he
Room service on speed dial was funny to see!

Amazing memories we made.

LOVING SUGGESTION #32

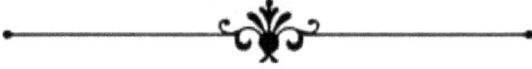

Always look for their favorite restaurants, so they look forward to the food.

DINING OUT

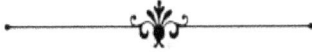

Footy like you, I have never seen
Dinning out so frequently
Thanks to you, I have tasted
The most delicious foods ever created

You are a magnificent treasure
Eating with you is such a pleasure
Always good and positive words spoken
I learned from you how to be unbroken

There is place in Copa Cabana
I've tasted the most delicious meats
Platters of steaks from every kind
When I saw that, it blew my mind

I'll take you there.

LOVING SUGGESTION #33

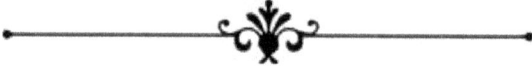

Massages are important for the body; they are also beneficial and relaxing. I pre-plan the massage appointments in advance.

MASSAGE TREATS

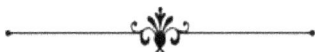

Looking forward to this day
I remind you days before it's time
Looking forward to replace
Anxiety and the stressful days

Feeling lovely and renewed
endorphins that boost your mood
Bonus is the facial massage
Awesome treat and a great wash

Smiley ladies, we had few laughs
What a day! We had a blast!

LOVING SUGGESTION #34

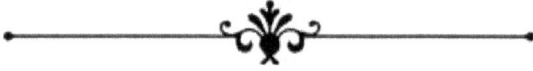

Many times, I asked my brother to join me for manicures and pedicures, we go every 3 weeks, and he loves getting his feet massaged and nails cleaned up.

FUN PAMPERING

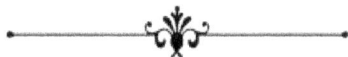

Grooming is another way
To get you out and enjoy your day
Exfoliation will do you good
Feeling pampered like you should

This is where you should stand
Wearing your sandals and walk the sand
Manicure will help you feel
Confident while eating your meal

Looking forward to this day

LOVING SUGGESTION #35

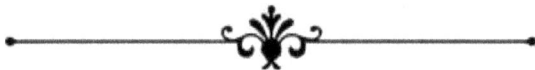

Try to include kids in your loved one's lives. Their innocent souls and beauty can light up their day.

PLAY DATES

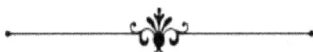

Planning play dates with your favorite boy
At times you are broken but still feel joy
My cousin told me that kids can heal
Wounded souls like yours, my dear

You never said no or declined my request
To be with him, you never are stressed
Eating pizza or shopping for toys
I hear pleasure in your excited voice

You always tell me that he is an art
For a 6-year-old that he is very smart
May God keep you alive to see
and be with him till eternity

Loving Suggestion #36

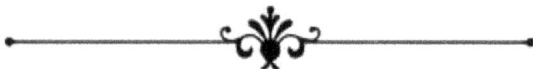

Holiday celebrations are important because of the spiritual strength it brings to all of us. Calendar and plan to have your loved one together with as many family members.

Special gifts can brighten their day. Create or buy something very special to brighten their room or the area they are spending most of their time in can be helpful.

Some examples: for the holidays, I wrote him a poem and attached a picture we took on a weekend trip. He felt special for taking my time to do that for him. He has it in his room, and it brings a smile to his face.

Another special gift I gave him is a radio cube from pastor Joel Osteen. He loves listening to him, and he plays his daily affirmations every morning.

Other examples include t-shirts from their favorite places, mugs, pajamas, bed sheets or pillows from their favorite name brands. They spend a lot of time at home so fill their place with happy memories and a lot of comfort.

SPECIAL GIFT
"THE HOLIDAYS POEM"

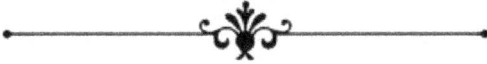

Dear Brother,

There is no blemish in your heart,
I just dislike when you randomly fart.
You are a pure joy to be around,
I treasure our moments on this ground.

You rose from the darkness like a full moon,
Happiness is waiting for you very soon.
Passport in your hand, and hello, Cancun,
Enjoying the sunshine on the lagoon.

I want you to make me a true promise,
Visualize your great life ahead of you.
Wake up and thank God for another day,
And recite the 4 prayers from our Prophet.

You are a child with a miraculous cure,
Because my brother, you are so pure.
God will find a way and keep you near,
And grow to old age with us each year.

LOVING SUGGESTION #37

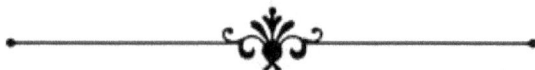

Birthday celebrations are important even if you don't normally celebrate it. Make plans for something special and talk about it with your family members. Write the birthday events and calendar them around any treatments your loved one has.

Since my brother's diagnosis, we have enhanced our birthday celebrations. I helped my brother shop for the gifts and also got him out of the house.

BIRTHDAY CELEBRATIONS

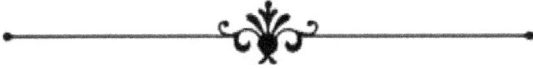

Birthday parties are special days
Looking forward to seeing our mom
Even on your darkest day
You have to find the gift today

There are times it's hard to shop
You give them cash or a gift card
Making your entrance, it's also hard
But being there is always a good start

Many times, you also say
That you forgot your own pain
And you are always glad you came
We thank you for your efforts

LOVING SUGGESTION #38

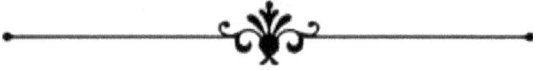

Take-out gatherings are important when your loved one doesn't feel like going out.

Invite some family members and suggest eating together. You can order or have each guest bring one item for everyone to enjoy.

TAKE OUT HAPPINESS

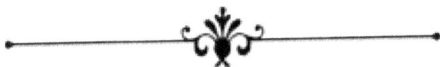

The days of your treatments,
Those are your resting days.
We gather to embrace you tight.
Yet another struggle and fight.

We order meals that you crave,
Foodie like you must be in the mood.
We laugh and enjoy gathering around you,
Not easy for what you are going through.

May you find an ease tomorrow.

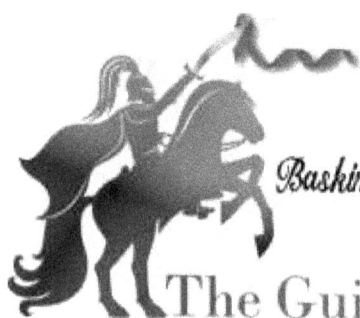

Bashim the Warrior

The Guiding Light

Chapter 6

BEFORE THE DIAGNOSIS

LOVING SUGGESTION #39

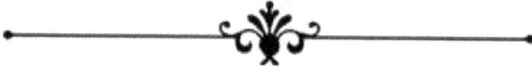

Please have your physicals each year, and when not feeling good, see a doctor immediately. If my brother did that, I don't think he would be in this situation and most likely not in stage 4.

———————— ❧ ————————

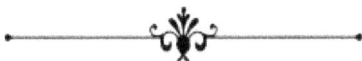

Baskim was born in a poetic town with a beautiful lake in Struga, Macedonia on July 11, 1975. He was the most handsome, vibrant, blonde boy that was so much fun. He was called a stud.

He had a beautiful childhood at the lake, with memories including learning to drive a car at the age of ten. He sold snails and watermelon to make his own money, out all-day swimming, playing basketball and soccer with his friends.

He was the youngest and my mom's favorite. He went with her everywhere. At the age of twelve, we all immigrated to America. He attended school until graduating high school and into working with my brother and father's construction business, and eventually joined the Union.

Baskim met the love of his life, Allison, at the age of 27. He knew it was his soulmate, and their love was a special one. When Allison was 25, she fell ill and was diagnosed with a rare disease known as Wegener's right before they were due to wed. He stayed to fight her illness for 15 years, but Allison died just months after Baskim was diagnosed with stage 4 lung cancer.

He loved her so much and worked so hard to get her health that he never cared for himself. That was one of the reasons I wanted to write this book. Seeing him put himself last and not being in his shoes to care for someone else. I know I had to make my own health a priority too. Please make sure you set your own physicals each year and follow up with your doctors when you feel something is wrong with your health. You can't take care of someone else if you can't take care of yourself.

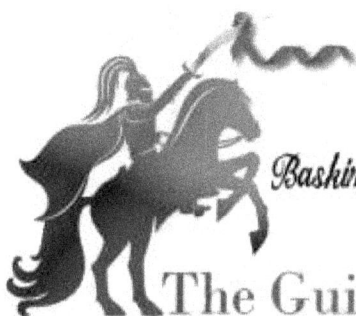

Bashim the Warrior

The Guiding Light

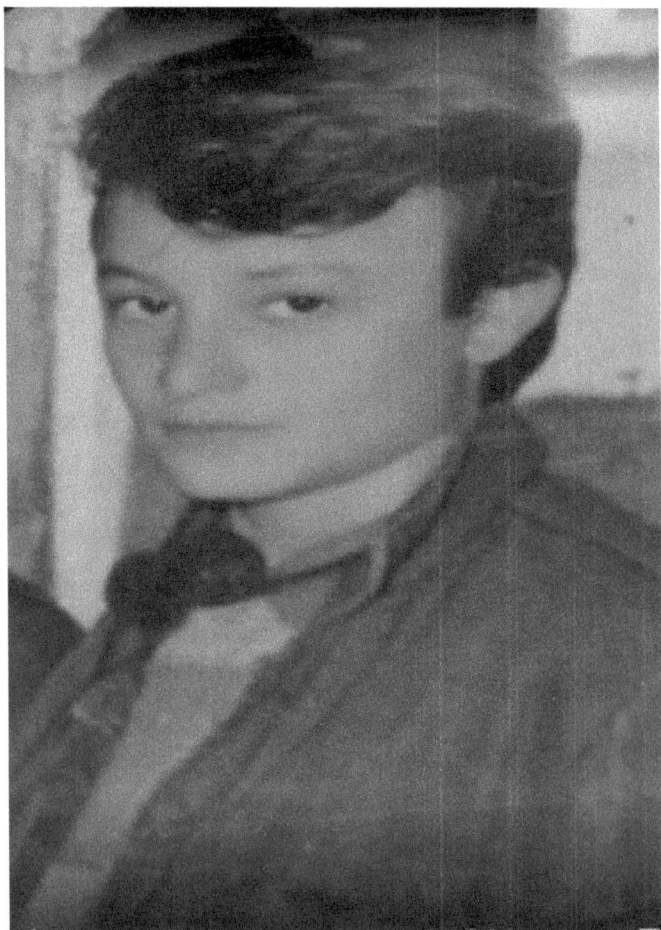

GOING DOWN MEMORY LANE

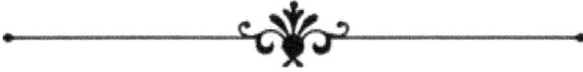

Full of Confidence

You grew up in a lake,
Swam and played each day.
The things that you would do,
Tall and handsome, you grew.

Always friends around you
Tricks that you would pull
Driving daddy's car
To show up like a star

Survivor from the start
As a small boy too smart
Selling stuff from a cart
With an amazing heart

Left the lovely land
What if we never came?
Will you go through this pain?
If not, we should have stayed.

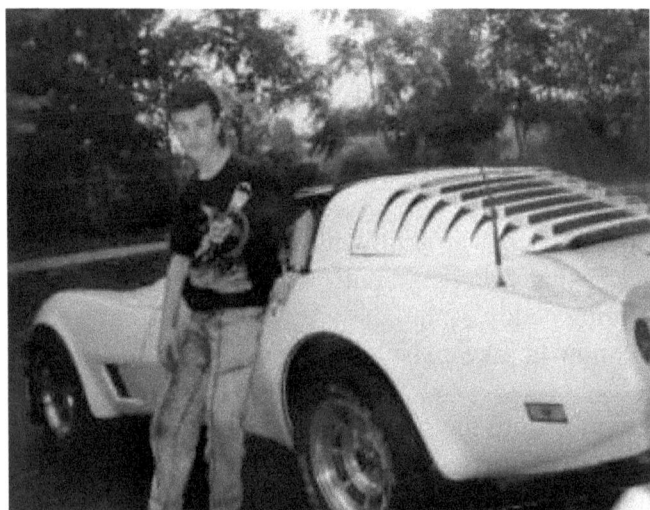

SCHOOL DAYS

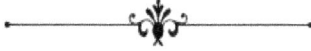

School was not your thing
Escaping as much as you could
Sneaking and hiding in the shed
And at times, under your bed

Your principal would knock
Neighbors dog will always bark
Funny moments with you
When he was looking for you

The most popular in school
Because you were so cool
Girls chased you everywhere
Always laughing and didn't care

You know you were the stud!

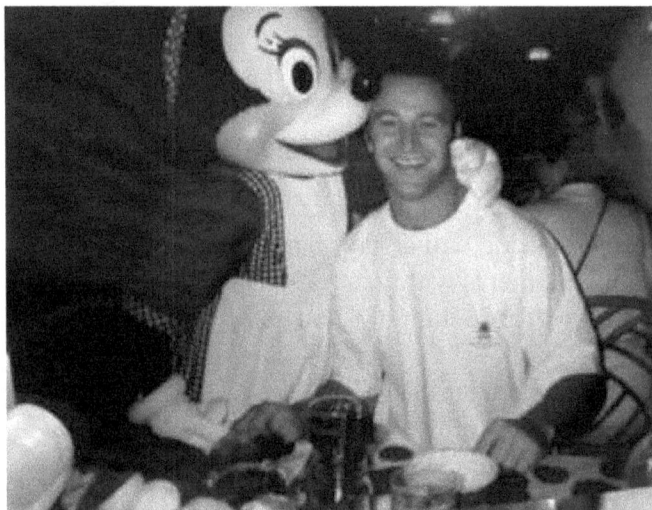

WHEN A YOUNG MAN

You were twenty-one
Waiting to hit the bar
Parties, friends and dancing
Always someone romancing

You were so neat and clean
Even ironed your jeans
Your bedroom was always locked
Angry when we had to knock

You met a lovely girl
Petite and smart from a far away land
You both were young; it had to end
A good thing you made her a friend

You were free to play again.

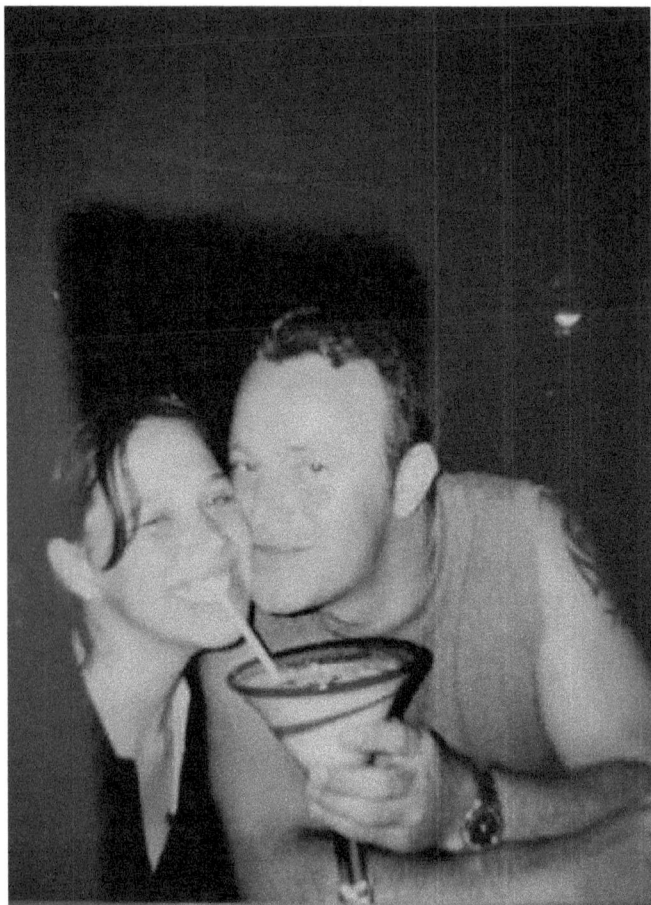

YOUR FOREVER LOVE

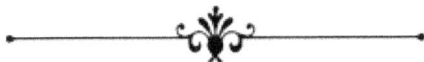

Once you met your girl
You said you found your pearl
Happy moments all the way
Hanging out every day

Trips around the USA
Vegas, Miami and LA
Dinners, parties and some more
A diamond ring was in store

Christmas parties, I came by
Amazing lady Allie's mom
Gave me gifts and never one
Now a true Angel from above

Left our house to live there
Calling no answer, what a scare
You called us back and said she is sick
Wegener's disease with two months to live.

You left us speechless…

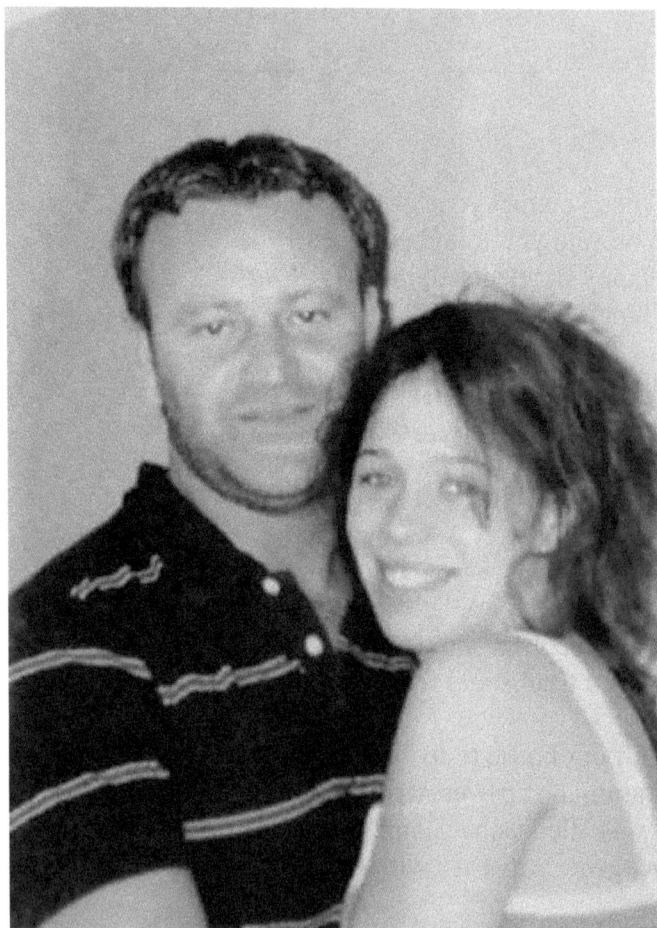

FIGHT FOR LOVE

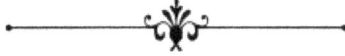

Love and pain in your face
Never seem to be amazed
How you took her illness
With your strong willingness

You took good care of her
Day and night by her side
She lived for you all the years
Cuddled together with no fears.

You walked on this ground
But we hardly saw you around
Not by choice but a hardship
Glad you felt her worship.

Lake Ohrid, Macedonia

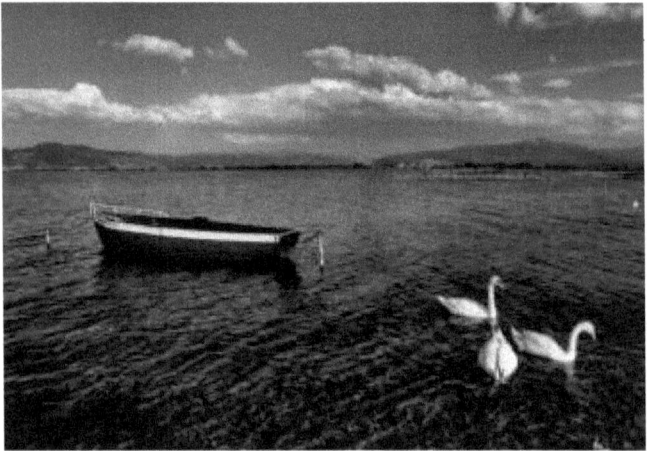

Photo by Slavica Panova

YOUR LOVE DIED

She left you. It's been a year
I know your love is not near
Left you weeping all alone
In the world of the unknown

You kept going…
Building the roads of construction
You are beating the enemy inside
With your strong family by your side

LOVING SUGGESTION #40

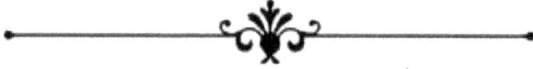

"Always give something special from your heart to people that help your loved one."

When my brother got diagnosed, the sister-in-law Jenny moved in to help her sister and my brother.

In the hardest of times, when his wife died, Jenny stayed and helped my brother with coping and healing. The Family is forever grateful for not leaving him alone while grieving his wife's passing. Jenny is part of our family.

I wrote this poem for Jenny as a Christmas present.

MY FRIEND JENNY

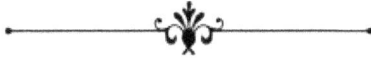

It's true. I never knew anyone like you…
So much passion and crazy things you do
Drinking coffee and talking things through
We make a power team, us two!

The heart of gold that you possess
Years of making for the world to impress
Your creative mind helped me address
Things about me that put me to stress

We laughed and cried every season
Heartbreak events left scars for a reasons
To grow and prosper and reach the sky
You are true warrior with a spirit to fly

Wish you a lifetime of joy and happiness
So much love and endless tenderness
And your land of making for you to reside
Grow life's nature with love by your side!

Thank you for helping my brother

The journey is better with you!

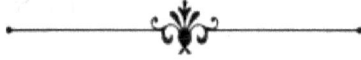

My sister-in-law Ness (my older brother's wife) helped me immensely throughout this journey, mentally as well as helping me with my son and cooking delicious meals for us.
She also helped by supplying and making gift baskets for anyone that helped my bother along the way.

"Forever, I will be grateful I never had a sister, but you are so close to it!

Ness, this poem is for you…

NESS'S ADDICTION TO COFFEE

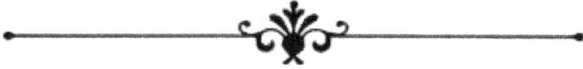

Fasting day is as a judgment day for some
All due to a liquid called "coffee."
She dreaded the days of its absence
Confused, walking without a balance

The morning rose, and so did the queen
Staring at the empty coffee machine
She said chuck full of nuts. It's my favorite
So, I savor it! Can't have it! Damn it!

———————— ❧ ————————

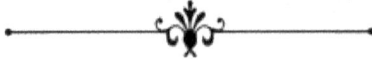

To the most beautiful and dearest niece Leyla, thank you for always helping in this journey, with my son, supplying gifts for people that helped Baskim along the way and all in between.

"A niece is so dear to your heart. If you never had a daughter, she feels so close to it."

This poem is for you beautiful…

BEAUTIFUL NIECE LEYLA

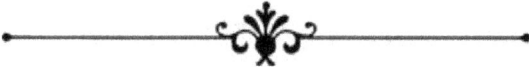

She is a dazzling princess ever since birth
Can't find a beauty like her on this earth
In all the kingdoms, the kings were waiting
The prince to hold her hand, anticipating

Leyla grew up happy and had at all
Strong family behind her to never let her fall
Always wore her crown and was very proud
The woman she is, applauded by a crowd

Mind like a wizard, executive job at her age
No man she chooses can compete at this stage
Fought for a woman's rights since she was a teen
Always disliked her parents' limiting belief

She didn't choose the prince but another
She has 2 best friends, her love and her brother
Happy, playful and loves music like her aunt
Working to open her lounge and find her content

She found her dream place, her gem
When you enter feels like a gentle autumn rain
As sweet as her future child playing violin
It's a place like you've never been!

Welcome to Leyla's Castle

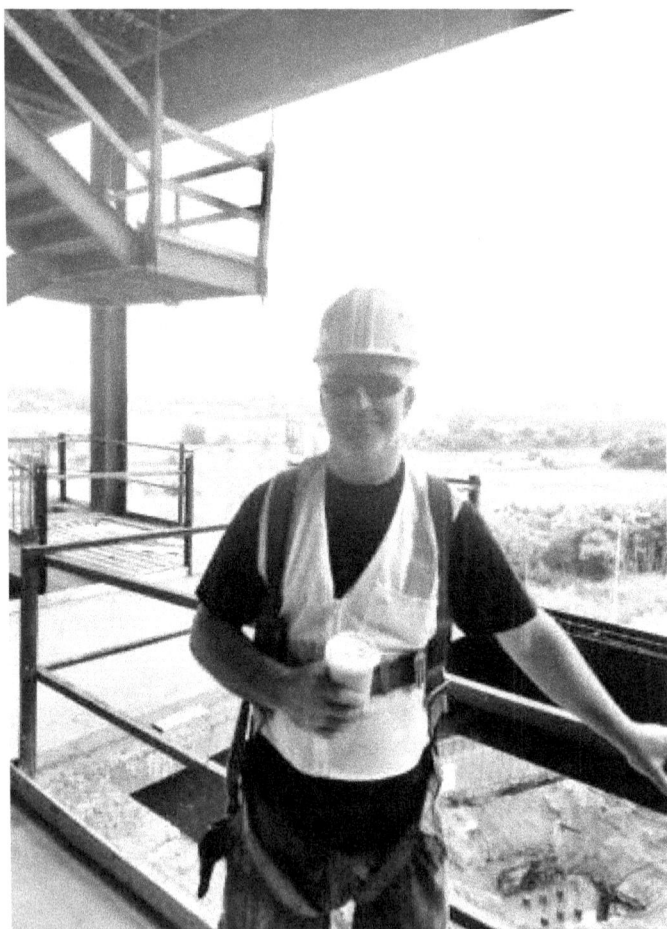

THE INTERVIEW WITH BASKIM

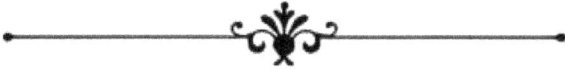

What do you want to tell the world?
I lived a great life.

What's your biggest accomplishment in life?
Working as a Mason. I am very proud of my work.

What was the happiest time in your life?
When I met Allie.

What's your biggest regret?
No regrets.

What hurt you the most?
When Allie died.

What would you do over again?
Nothing

Where from here?
To be healthy, not to feel sick.

What do you wish to happen?
Your book to be successful, having my family is what's important to me. I also wish for the pain to go away.

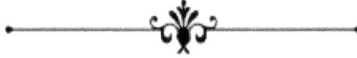

"Fulfilling wishes of your loved one will bring you so much joy in your soul and give them a reason to dream again."

Chapter 7

HIS WISH -VISITING MOTHERLAND MACEDONIA

Lake Ohrid, Macedonia

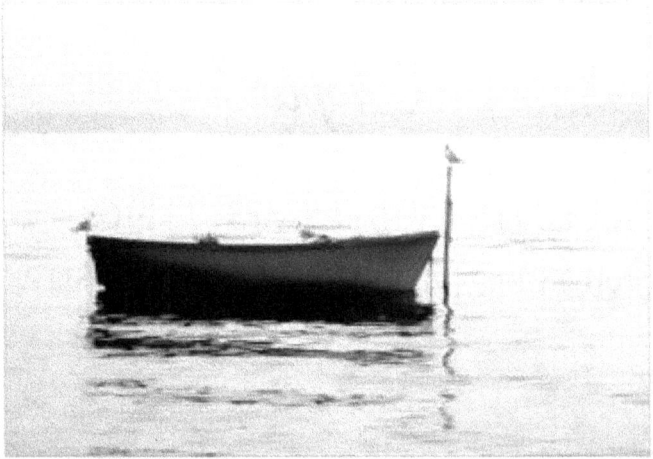

Photo by Slavica Panova

———————— ❦ ————————

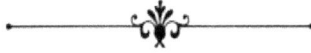

Baskim has not visited Macedonia since he left 34 years ago. His wish is to go back in August 2022 for 3 weeks. Most of the family that lives overseas are in Switzerland, Italy, and Belgium and will be there vacationing at that time. There is a first cousin's wedding we are invited to. Family will be traveling along with Baskim. We are all so excited about this trip and the family in Macedonia is so happy and anticipating his arrival. We can't wait to make new memories.

Grni Drim,Struga, Macedonia

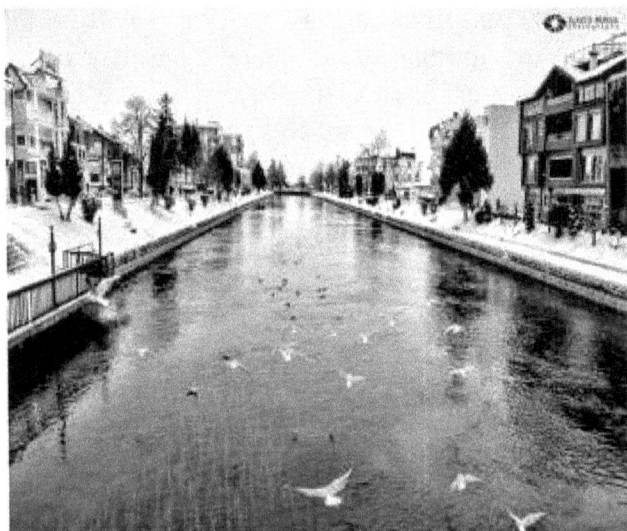

Photo by Slavica Panova

FULFILLING YOUR WISH

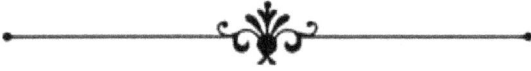

You came to this dreamland at twelve
Missed your homeland but never went back
Family calling from around the globe
To see you and hug your amazing soul

You are determined to go back and see
The beautiful lake and drink mountain tea
Making plans when its sunny and bright
Sit in a café and watch people at night

Anticipating great August summer days
Our family and friends will be amazed
Of your incredible grace, you will be praised
Motherland, open your arms
He is coming...

Lake Ohrid, Macedonia

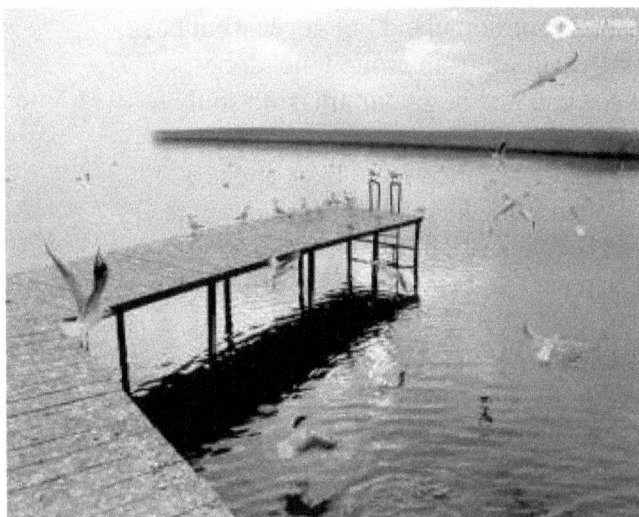

Photo by Slavica Panova

ASKING YOU

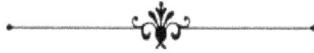

Oh, dear friends and family
Be gentle and kind when you greet him
Don't accuse and be offended by his absence
With a destiny as his, it was hard for him to balance

Oh, dear friends and family
Don't be afraid to ask him about his journey
And don't treat him as a patient
He is aware and smart; he won't fall apart

Oh, dear friends and family
Please come by to visit and invite
Let's all enjoy together day and night
Make happy memories and his trip light!

Thank you in advance.

Poetry Night, Struga, Macedonia

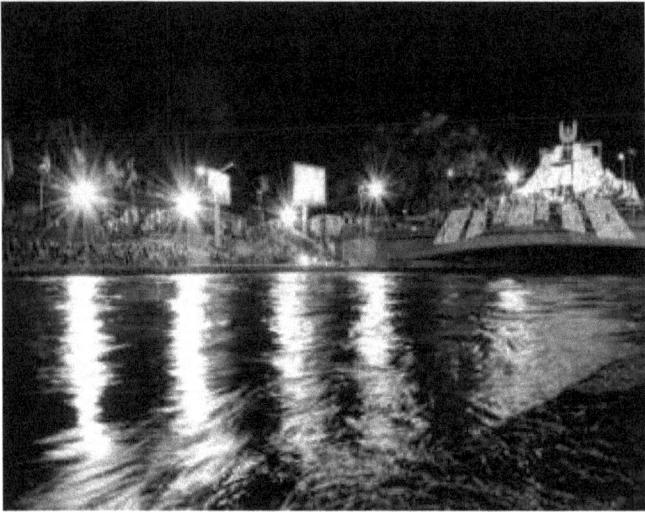

Photo by Slavica Panova

MY POETRY TOWN STRUGA

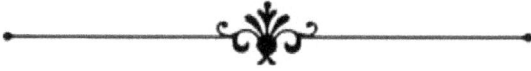

You hold in your palms the most beautiful lake
And black river that runs through your veins
When I think of you, my darkness, you drain
Traveling to you feels like there is no more rain

The August month shines in magical poetry nights
Festival for all with all sorts of lights and bites
How I long for those nights to be near
With my best friend to recite our poetry each year.

Macedonian dessert "Indijanka"

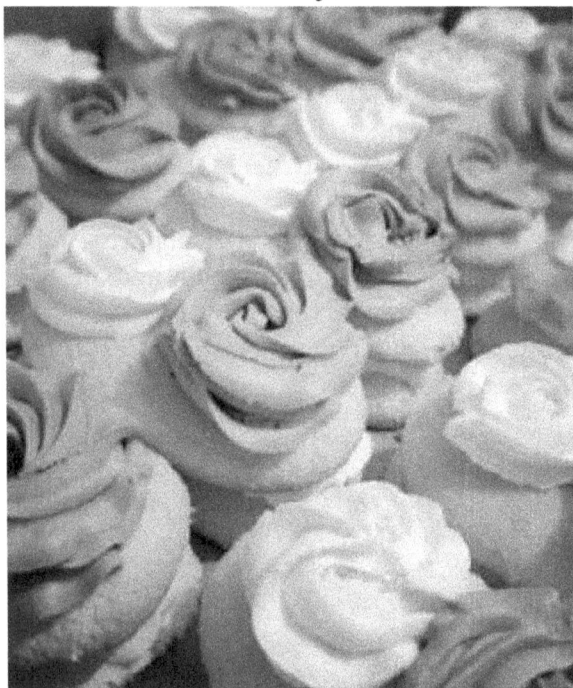

Photo and made by Chef Nirgul Abdula

LOVE FOR YOUR FOOD

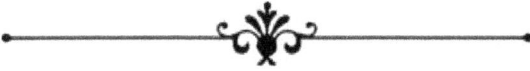

We will come to you as soon as he awakes
Relax at the cafe and eat his Indianka cake
And the tastiest hamburgers inside with fries
All delicious organic foods, it's no surprise

Those two things left in his memory
But I haven't been a stranger to you
I embrace you and feel for all my people
Love all the languages you speak of

You eat the most delicious food on this earth
And your warmest culture I've seen since birth
Have us as your guest and say no more
We will be grateful forevermore

Struga, Macedonia

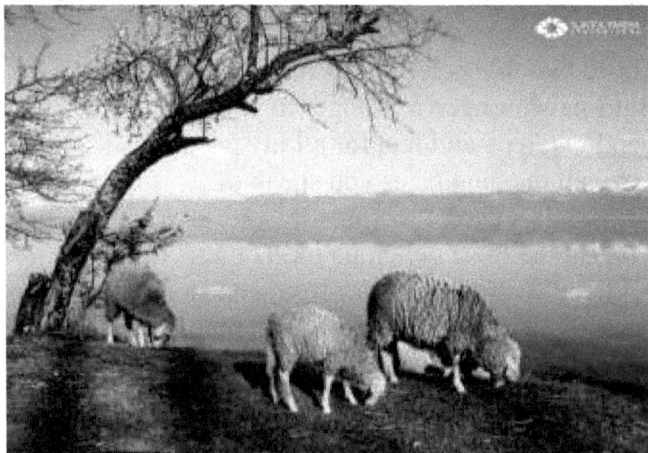

Photo by Slavica Panova

OH MOTHERLAND

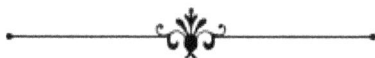

When he arrives and places his feet on your soil,
Hug him tight and wrap him in magical light.
So bright and cleanse his soul inside,
Bring him back to when he was an innocent boy

Can't bear to see our lives so shattered,
Please help us as I have always loved you.
Create a miraculous cure when he is there,
And invite your entire country to a prayer

Blessings to your land and all your people!

TO BE CONTINUED ...

FAMILY PHOTO

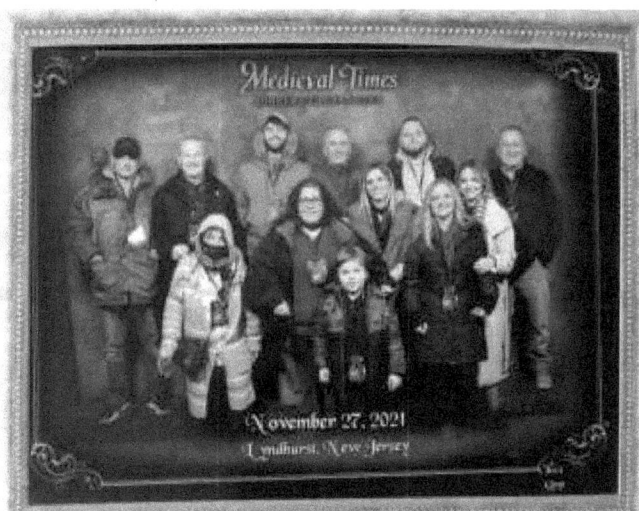

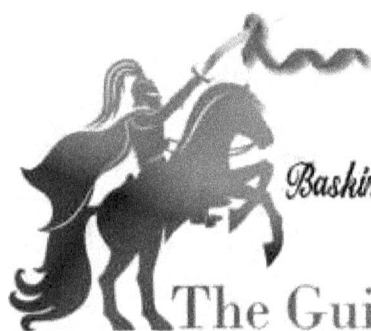

Bashim the Warrior

The Guiding Light

DEEPEST GRATITUDE

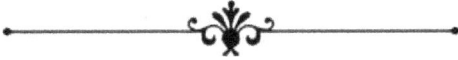

I would like to send a very special thank you to the team at St. Joseph's Hospital in Wayne, NJ. The array of people we encountered here can only be described as knowing the true meaning of humanity. Their caring, empathy and their ability to comfort their patients are truly a miracle. Special thanks go to: Dr Dorkhom, Dr Nabulsi, CCU team, the surgical team, Angela, Leah, Naser, Anabel, Ruki, Etem, Liz, Kadesha, Gulten, Bianca, Cynthia, Katerine. Every single one of you has made a positive and everlasting imprint on my family and me. You've taken a situation that is almost impossible to navigate and made the road a little smoother. I could never thank you enough. I am forever in your debt.

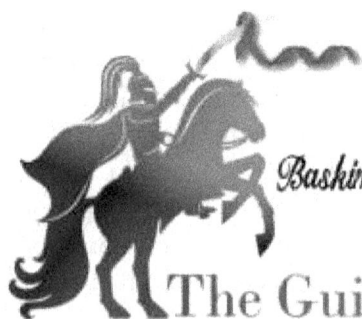

Baskim the Warrior

The Guiding Light

ABOUT THE AUTHOR

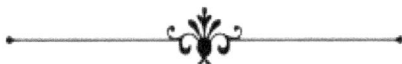

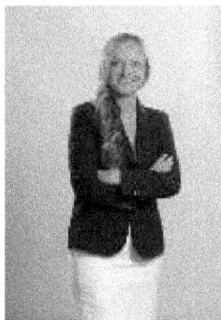

Zana Kenjar is a leadership consultant, publishing mentor, and founder of ZK Publishing House. After two decades of leading teams in the corporate world, she now dedicates her time to helping others share their stories and build meaningful legacies through books.

She is the author of the international bestseller *Becoming a Legacy Leader* and *Standing Together Against Cancer*, both written with deep intention and compassion. Her personal journey marked by faith, healing, and devotion to family continues to shape her coaching and writing.

Born in Macedonia and now living in New Jersey with her husband and son, Zana is proud to share her work in both English and Macedonian. She believes in the power of prayer, storytelling, and uplifting others to live with purpose and courage.

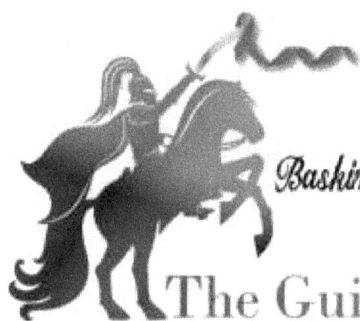

Bashin the Warrior

The Guiding Light

THANK YOU

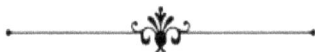

I would personally like to thank you for purchasing and investing your time in reading this book.
Please share it with your friends and family or purchase it for a loved one that you think will benefit.

Your input is very valuable. If you received value from this book, please leave me a helpful review on Amazon, letting me and others know what you thought about this book.

Praying for your health, love and prosperity!

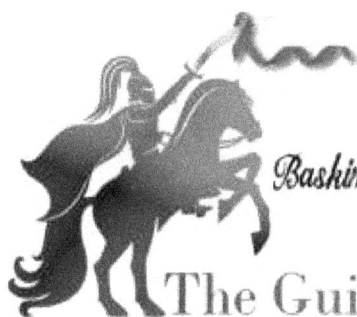

Bashim the Warrior

The Guiding Light